Zero Point Grilled Recipes for Weight Loss

Deliciously, Healthy Outdoor Cooking for Shedding Pounds and Savoring Flavor to Ignite Your Weight Loss Journey and Enhance Vibrant Lifestyle.

DR. HELENA M. OLIVIA

Copyright Page

Copyright © [2023] by Dr. Helena M. Olivia All rights reserved. No part of this publication may be reproduced, distributed, or transmitted in any form or by any means, including photocopying, recording or other electronic or mechanical methods, without the prior written permission of the publisher, except in the case of brief quotations embodied in critical reviews and certain other noncommercial uses permitted by copyright law.

TABLE OF CONTENTS

Concept of Zero Point Foods	4
Benefits of Zero Point Foods for Weight Loss	6
Grilled Lemon Herb Chicken Breast	8
Balsamic Grilled Vegetables	10
Grilled Shrimp Skewers	12
Grilled Salmon with Dill	14
Grilled Chicken Caesar Salad	16
Spicy Grilled Shrimp Skewers	18
Grilled Turkey Burgers	20
Grilled Portobello Mushrooms	22
Grilled Zucchini Planks	24
Grilled Garlic Lime Chicken	26
Grilled Tuna Steaks	28
Grilled Asparagus Spears	30
Grilled Cauliflower Steaks	32
Grilled Swordfish with Herb Butter	34
Grilled Eggplant Slices	36
Grilled Chicken and Veggie Kabobs	38
Grilled Mahi Mahi with Mango Salsa	40
Grilled Bell Pepper Rings	42
Grilled Turkey Sausages	44
Grilled Bruschetta Chicken	46
Grilled Radicchio Wedges	48

Grilled Chicken Fajitas	50
Grilled Fish Tacos	52
Grilled Pork Tenderloin	54
Grilled Caprese Chicken	56
Grilled Tilapia with Lemon Butter	58
Grilled Greek Chicken Souvlaki	60
Grilled Cabbage Wedges	62
Grilled Teriyaki Tofu	64
Grilled Vegetable Quesadillas	66
Grilled Vegetable Platter with Hummus	68
Grilled Spicy Tofu	70
Grilled Buffalo Cauliflower	72
30-Day Meal Plan	74
Zero Point Food List	76

CONCEPT OF ZERO POINT FOODS

Zero Point Foods are foods that have a low or zero SmartPoints value in certain diet programs. These programs assign points to different foods based on their nutritional content. The idea behind Zero Point Foods is that you can enjoy these foods without having to count their points towards your daily allowance. The specific Zero Point Foods can vary depending on the diet program you're following. Usually, these foods are low in calories and high in nutrients, like fruits, vegetables, lean proteins, and whole grains. Since they are lower in calories, you can eat them in larger quantities without worrying about going over your daily points. Including Zero Point Foods in your meals and snacks can help you feel satisfied while staying on track with your goals. They provide a great opportunity to make healthier choices and incorporate more nutritious options into your diet.

- **Weight Loss Programs:** Zero point foods are commonly featured in weight loss programs that utilize a points-based system to help individuals track their food intake. These programs assign points to different foods based on their nutritional content, with the goal of encouraging healthier eating habits and portion control.

- **Zero Point Value:** Foods designated as zero point foods are given a point value of zero, meaning individuals can consume them without counting them towards their daily point allowance. This encourages the consumption of these foods as part of a balanced diet.

- Nutrient Density: Zero point foods are typically nutrient-dense, meaning they provide a high amount of nutrients relative to their calorie content. These foods often include fruits, vegetables, lean proteins, and certain whole grains. By focusing on these foods, individuals can increase their intake of essential vitamins, minerals, and fiber while keeping their calorie intake in check.

- Portion Control: While zero point foods may be assigned zero points, portion control is still important. Consuming excessive amounts of these foods can still contribute to weight gain. Weight loss programs often provide guidance on portion sizes to help individuals make informed choices about their food intake.

- Flexibility: Zero point foods offer flexibility within the program, allowing individuals to build meals and snacks around these foods without feeling restricted. This flexibility can help individuals adhere to their dietary goals over the long term and maintain a balanced and sustainable approach to eating.

BENEFITS OF ZERO POINT FOODS FOR WEIGHT LOSS

- **Low in Calories:** Zero point foods are typically low in calories, which means you can consume them in larger quantities without significantly increasing your overall calorie intake. This can help you feel satisfied and full while still adhering to a calorie deficit, which is necessary for weight loss.

- **High in Nutrients:** Despite being low in calories, zero point foods are often rich in essential nutrients such as vitamins, minerals, and antioxidants. Consuming a variety of nutrient-dense foods supports overall health and well-being, ensuring you get the necessary nutrients while cutting calories for weight loss.

- **Promotes Satiety:** Many zero point foods are high in fiber, water, and protein, all of which contribute to feelings of fullness and satiety. By incorporating these foods into your meals, you can help control hunger and cravings, making it easier to stick to your weight loss plan without feeling deprived.

- **Encourages Healthy Eating Habits:** By focusing on these foods, you naturally reduce your intake of less healthy options like processed foods, sugary snacks, and high-fat foods, promoting a healthier overall diet.

- **Flexibility and Variety:** Zero point foods offer flexibility in meal planning and allow for a wide variety of food choices. This can help prevent boredom with your diet and make it easier to stick to your weight loss goals in the long term.

- **Supports Sustainable Weight Loss:** Because zero point foods are nutritious, filling, and satisfying, they support sustainable weight loss by providing a foundation for a balanced and enjoyable eating plan.

- **Blood Sugar Control:** Foods like non-starchy vegetables and lean proteins have minimal impact on blood sugar levels, which is beneficial for individuals with diabetes or those looking to stabilize their blood sugar levels.

GRILLED LEMON HERB CHICKEN BREAST

Prep Time 40 Mins

Cook Time 16 Mins

Yields 4 Servings

Prep Time including marinating

INGREDIENTS

- 4 boneless, skinless chicken breasts
- Juice of 2 lemons
- Zest of 1 lemon
- 2 cloves garlic, minced
- 2 tablespoons fresh chopped herbs (such as parsley, thyme, or rosemary)
- Salt and pepper to taste

DIRECTIONS

- In a small bowl, combine the lemon juice, lemon zest, minced garlic, and chopped herbs. Mix well.
- Place the chicken breasts in a shallow dish or large resealable plastic bag. Pour the lemon herb marinade over the chicken, making sure it's evenly coated. Marinate in the refrigerator for at least 30 minutes, or up to 4 hours.
- Preheat the grill to medium-high heat.
- Remove the chicken from the marinade and discard any excess marinade.

NUTRITIONAL FACTS (PER SERVING)

- Calories: 165kcal
- Total Fat: 3g
- Saturated Fat: 1g
- Cholesterol: 73mg
- Sodium: 77mg
- Carbohydrates: 2g
- Dietary Fiber: 0g
- Sugars: 0g
- Protein: 31g

DIRECTIONS

- Season the chicken breasts with salt and pepper on both sides.
- Place the chicken breasts on the preheated grill and cook for 6-8 minutes per side, or until the chicken is cooked through and no longer pink in the center. The internal temperature should reach 165°F (75°C).
- Remove the chicken from the grill and let it rest for a few minutes before serving.

BALSAMIC GRILLED VEGETABLES

Prep Time 10 Mins

Cook Time 15 Mins

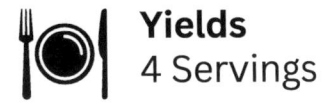

Yields 4 Servings

INGREDIENTS

- Assorted vegetables of your choice (such as bell peppers, zucchini, mushrooms, onions, cherry tomatoes, eggplant, etc.), sliced or chopped
- 2-3 tablespoons balsamic vinegar
- 1-2 cloves garlic, minced
- 1-2 tablespoons olive oil (optional)
- Salt and pepper to taste
- Fresh herbs (such as basil, thyme, or rosemary), chopped (optional)

DIRECTIONS

- Preheat your grill to medium-high heat.
- In a large bowl, combine the balsamic vinegar, minced garlic, olive oil (if using), salt, and pepper. Whisk until well combined.
- Add the sliced/chopped vegetables to the bowl with the balsamic marinade. Toss until the vegetables are evenly coated.
- If you have time, let the vegetables marinate for about 15-30 minutes to allow the flavors to meld.
- Once the grill is hot, place the marinated vegetables directly on the grill grates.

NUTRITIONAL FACTS (PER SERVING)

- Calories: 50kcal
- Total Fat: 1g
- Saturated Fat: 0g
- Cholesterol: 0mg
- Sodium: 5mg
- Carbohydrates: 10g
- Dietary Fiber: 3g
- Sugars: 5g
- Protein: 2g

DIRECTIONS

- You can use a grilling basket or skewers for smaller vegetables to prevent them from falling through the grates.
- Grill the vegetables for about 5-7 minutes per side, or until they are tender and have grill marks.
- Remove the grilled vegetables from the grill and transfer them to a serving platter. Sprinkle with fresh herbs if desired.
- Serve immediately and enjoy your delicious balsamic grilled vegetables!

GRILLED SHRIMP SKEWERS

Prep Time 10 Mins
Cook Time 8 Mins
Yields 4 Servings

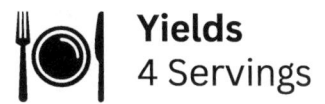

Marinating Time: 15 Mins

INGREDIENTS

- 1 lb large shrimp, peeled and deveined
- 2 cloves garlic, minced
- 2 tbsp fresh lemon juice
- 1 tbsp olive oil
- 1 tsp paprika
- Salt and pepper to taste
- Metal or wooden skewers, soaked in water if using wooden ones
- Optional: chopped fresh herbs such as parsley or cilantro for garnish.

DIRECTIONS

- In a blender, combine cucumbers, bell pepper, onion, garlic, red wine vinegar, lemon juice, salt, and pepper. Blend until smooth.
- Add Greek yogurt, dill, and parsley. Blend again until well combined.
- Gradually add vegetable broth until desired consistency is reached. Blend until smooth.
- Taste and adjust seasoning if necessary.
- Refrigerate for at least 2 hours before serving to allow flavors to meld.
- Serve chilled, garnished with additional fresh herbs if desired.

**NUTRITIONAL FACTS
(PER SERVING)**

- Calories: 120kcal
- Total Fat: 3g
- Saturated Fat: 0.5g
- Cholesterol: 215mg
- Sodium: 220mg
- Carbohydrates: 2g
- Dietary Fiber: 0g
- Sugars: 0g
- Protein: 22g

GRILLED SALMON WITH DILL

Prep Time 5 Mins

Cook Time 10 Mins

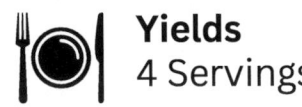

Yields 4 Servings

INGREDIENTS

- 4 salmon fillets (about 6 ounces each)
- 2 tablespoons chopped fresh dill
- 2 tablespoons lemon juice
- Salt and pepper to taste
- Lemon wedges for serving (optional)

DIRECTIONS

- Preheat your grill to medium-high heat.
- In a small bowl, mix together the chopped dill and lemon juice.
- Season the salmon fillets with salt and pepper to taste.
- Brush the dill and lemon mixture onto both sides of the salmon fillets.
- Place the salmon fillets on the preheated grill and cook for about 4-5 minutes per side, or until the salmon is cooked through and easily flakes with a fork.
- Remove the salmon from the grill and serve hot with lemon wedges if desired.

NUTRITIONAL FACTS (PER SERVING)

- Calories: 230kcal
- Total Fat: 11g
- Saturated Fat: 2g
- Cholesterol: 80mg
- Sodium: 70mg
- Carbohydrates: 0g
- Dietary Fiber: 0g
- Sugars: 0g
- Protein: 31g

GRILLED CHICKEN CAESAR SALAD

Prep Time
10 Mins

Cook Time
15 Mins

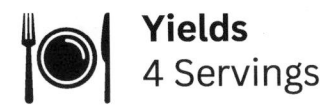

Yields
4 Servings

INGREDIENTS

- 4 boneless, skinless chicken breasts
- Salt and pepper, to taste
- 1 tablespoon olive oil
- 1 head romaine lettuce, washed and chopped
- 1/4 cup grated Parmesan cheese
- Caesar salad dressing (use a low-fat or homemade version for fewer points)
- Optional: Croutons (consider using whole grain for fewer points)

DIRECTIONS

- Preheat grill to medium-high heat.
- Season chicken breasts with salt, pepper, and olive oil.
- Grill chicken for about 6-7 minutes per side, or until cooked through (internal temperature of 165°F or 75°C).
- Remove chicken from grill and let it rest for a few minutes before slicing.

Salad Assembly:

- In a large bowl, toss chopped romaine lettuce with grated Parmesan cheese.
- Divide the lettuce among 4 plates.
- Top each plate with sliced grilled chicken.

NUTRITIONAL FACTS (PER SERVING)

- Calories: 180kcal
- Protein: 30g
- Fat: 5g
- Carbohydrates: 3g
- Fiber: 2g

DIRECTIONS

- Drizzle Caesar dressing over the salads according to your preference.
- If desired, sprinkle with croutons.

SPICY GRILLED SHRIMP SKEWERS

Prep Time
20 Mins

Cook Time
8 Mins

Yields
4 Servings

INGREDIENTS

- 1 lb large shrimp, peeled and deveined
- 2 cloves garlic, minced
- 1 tablespoon olive oil
- 1 teaspoon paprika
- 1/2 teaspoon cayenne pepper (adjust according to your spice preference)
- 1/2 teaspoon black pepper
- 1/2 teaspoon salt
- 1 tablespoon fresh parsley, chopped (for garnish)
- Lemon wedges (for serving)

DIRECTIONS

- If you're using wooden skewers, soak them in water for about 30 minutes to prevent burning.
- In a bowl, mix together minced garlic, olive oil, paprika, cayenne pepper, black pepper, and salt.
- Add the shrimp to the bowl and toss until they are evenly coated with the spice mixture. Allow the shrimp to marinate for at least 15 minutes.
- Preheat your grill to medium-high heat.
- Thread the shrimp onto the skewers, distributing them evenly.

NUTRITIONAL FACTS (PER SERVING)

- Calories: 150kcal
- Protein: 24g
- Fat: 4g
- Carbohydrates: 2g
- Fiber: 0.5g
- Sodium: 380mg

DIRECTIONS

- Place the skewers on the grill and cook for about 2-3 minutes per side, or until the shrimp are pink and opaque.
- Once cooked, remove the skewers from the grill and garnish with chopped parsley.
- Serve hot with lemon wedges on the side.

GRILLED TURKEY BURGERS

Prep Time
10 Mins

Cook Time
12 Mins

Yields
4 Servings

INGREDIENTS

- 1 lb lean ground turkey (preferably 93% lean)
- 1/4 cup finely chopped onion
- 2 cloves garlic, minced
- 1 tsp Worcestershire sauce
- 1 tsp Dijon mustard
- 1/2 tsp salt
- 1/4 tsp black pepper
- Cooking spray for greasing the grill

DIRECTIONS

- Preheat your grill to medium-high heat.
- In a large mixing bowl, combine the ground turkey, chopped onion, minced garlic, Worcestershire sauce, Dijon mustard, salt, and black pepper. Mix until all ingredients are evenly distributed.
- Divide the mixture into 4 equal portions and shape each portion into a patty.
- Lightly coat the grill grates with cooking spray to prevent sticking.
- Place the turkey burger patties on the preheated grill and cook for 5-6 minutes on each side, or until the internal temperature reaches 165°F (75°C) and the burgers are cooked through.

NUTRITIONAL FACTS (PER SERVING)

- Calories: 45kcal
- Total Fat: 7g
- Saturated Fat: 2g
- Cholesterol: 80mg
- Sodium: 320mg
- Carbohydrates: 2g
- Dietary Fiber: 0g
- Sugars: 1g
- Protein: 20g

DIRECTIONS

- Once cooked, remove the burgers from the grill and let them rest for a few minutes before serving.

GRILLED PORTOBELLO MUSHROOMS

Prep Time
35 Mins

Cook Time
10 Mins

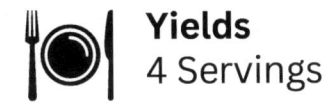

Yields
4 Servings

INGREDIENTS

- 4 large portobello mushrooms
- 2 cloves garlic, minced
- 2 tablespoons balsamic vinegar
- 2 tablespoons low-sodium soy sauce
- 1 tablespoon olive oil
- Salt and pepper to taste
- Fresh herbs (optional), such as parsley or thyme, for garnish

DIRECTIONS

- Clean the portobello mushrooms by wiping them with a damp cloth or paper towel to remove any dirt. Remove the stems and discard or reserve for another use.
- In a small bowl, whisk together the minced garlic, balsamic vinegar, low-sodium soy sauce, and olive oil to make the marinade.
- Place the cleaned mushrooms in a shallow dish or a resealable plastic bag. Pour the marinade over the mushrooms, making sure they are evenly coated. Marinate for at least 30 minutes, turning occasionally to ensure all sides are coated.

NUTRITIONAL FACTS (PER SERVING)

- Calories: 45kcal
- Total Fat: 2g
- Sodium: 235mg
- Carbohydrates: 5g
- Dietary Fiber: 2g
- Sugars: 2g
- Protein: 3g

DIRECTIONS

- Preheat the grill to medium-high heat.
- Remove the mushrooms from the marinade and shake off any excess. Season with salt and pepper to taste.
- Place the mushrooms on the preheated grill, gill side down. Grill for 4-5 minutes on each side, or until the mushrooms are tender and have grill marks.
- Once grilled, remove the mushrooms from the grill and let them rest for a few minutes.
- Garnish with fresh herbs, if desired, before serving.

GRILLED ZUCCHINI PLANKS

Prep Time
5 Mins

Cook Time
10 Mins

Yields
4 Servings

INGREDIENTS

- 4 medium zucchinis, washed and sliced lengthwise into planks
- Cooking spray
- Salt and pepper to taste
- Optional: your choice of herbs or spices such as garlic powder, onion powder, or Italian seasoning

DIRECTIONS

- Preheat your grill to medium-high heat.
- Spray the zucchini planks lightly with cooking spray on both sides.
- Season the zucchini planks with salt, pepper, and any desired herbs or spices.
- Place the zucchini planks directly on the grill grates.
- Grill the zucchini planks for about 3-4 minutes on each side, or until they are tender and have grill marks.
- Once cooked, remove the zucchini planks from the grill and serve hot.

**NUTRITIONAL FACTS
(PER SERVING)**

- Calories: 18kcal
- Total Fat: 0.4g
- Sodium: 3mg
- Carbohydrates: 3.6g
- Dietary Fiber: 1.3g
- Sugars: 2.3g
- Protein: 1.3g

GRILLED GARLIC LIME CHICKEN

Prep Time
35 Mins
including Marinating

Cook Time
16 Mins

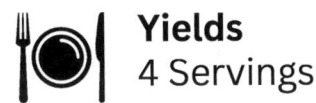

Yields
4 Servings

INGREDIENTS

- 4 boneless, skinless chicken breasts
- 4 cloves garlic, minced
- Zest and juice of 2 limes
- 2 tablespoons chopped fresh cilantro
- Salt and pepper, to taste

DIRECTIONS

- In a small bowl, combine the minced garlic, lime zest, lime juice, chopped cilantro, salt, and pepper to create the marinade.
- Place the chicken breasts in a shallow dish or a resealable plastic bag. Pour the marinade over the chicken, making sure each piece is well coated. Marinate in the refrigerator for at least 30 minutes, or up to 4 hours.
- Preheat the grill to medium-high heat.
- Remove the chicken from the marinade, shaking off any excess, and discard the remaining marinade.

NUTRITIONAL FACTS (PER SERVING)

- Calories: 160kcal
- Total Fat: 3g
- Saturated Fat: 1g
- Cholesterol: 73mg
- Sodium: 68mg
- Carbohydrates: 2g
- Dietary Fiber: 0g
- Sugars: 0g
- Protein: 30g

DIRECTIONS

- Grill the chicken breasts for 6-8 minutes on each side, or until they are cooked through and no longer pink in the center. The internal temperature should reach 165°F (75°C).
- Once cooked, remove the chicken from the grill and let it rest for a few minutes before serving.
- Serve the grilled garlic lime chicken with your favorite side dishes or as part of a salad.

GRILLED TUNA STEAKS

Prep Time 10 Mins **Cook Time** 8 Mins **Yields** 4 Servings

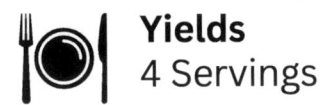

INGREDIENTS

- 4 tuna steaks, about 6 ounces each
- 2 tablespoons olive oil
- 2 cloves garlic, minced
- 2 teaspoons lemon zest
- 2 tablespoons lemon juice
- 1 teaspoon dried oregano
- Salt and pepper to taste
- Lemon wedges for serving
- Chopped parsley for garnish (optional)

DIRECTIONS

- Preheat your grill to medium-high heat.
- In a small bowl, whisk together the olive oil, minced garlic, lemon zest, lemon juice, dried oregano, salt, and pepper to create a marinade.
- Place the tuna steaks in a shallow dish and pour the marinade over them, turning to coat evenly. Let them marinate for about 15-20 minutes while the grill heats up.
- Once the grill is hot, place the tuna steaks on the grill grates. Grill for about 3-4 minutes on each side, or until desired doneness. For medium-rare, the internal temperature should reach 125°F (52°C).

NUTRITIONAL FACTS (PER SERVING)

- Calories: 220kcal
- Total Fat: 10g
- Saturated Fat: 2g
- Cholesterol: 85mg
- Sodium: 85mg
- Carbohydrates: 1g
- Dietary Fiber: 0g
- Sugars: 0g
- Protein: 31g

DIRECTIONS

- Remove the tuna steaks from the grill and let them rest for a few minutes before serving.
- Garnish with chopped parsley and serve with lemon wedges on the side.

GRILLED ASPARAGUS SPEARS

Prep Time 5 Mins

Cook Time 7 Mins

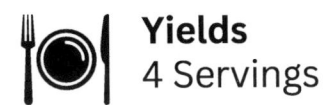

Yields 4 Servings

INGREDIENTS

- 1 bunch of asparagus spears, tough ends trimmed
- 1 tablespoon olive oil
- Salt and pepper to taste
- Lemon wedges for serving (optional)

DIRECTIONS

- Preheat your grill to medium-high heat.
- In a large bowl, toss the asparagus spears with olive oil until evenly coated.
- Season the asparagus with salt and pepper to taste.
- Place the asparagus spears directly on the grill grate, perpendicular to the grates, to prevent them from falling through.
- Grill the asparagus for 5-7 minutes, turning occasionally, until they are tender and slightly charred.
- Remove the grilled asparagus from the grill and transfer to a serving platter.

NUTRITIONAL FACTS (PER SERVING)

- Calories: 35kcal
- Total Fat: 2g
- Saturated Fat: 0g
- Cholesterol: 0mg
- Sodium: 0mg
- Carbohydrates: 4g
- Dietary Fiber: 2g
- Sugars: 2g
- Protein: 2g

DIRECTIONS

- Squeeze fresh lemon juice over the grilled asparagus before serving, if desired.

GRILLED CAULIFLOWER STEAKS

Prep Time
10 Mins

Cook Time
12 Mins

Yields
3 Servings

INGREDIENTS

- 1 head cauliflower
- 2 tablespoons olive oil
- 2 cloves garlic, minced
- 1 teaspoon paprika
- 1/2 teaspoon cumin
- Salt and pepper to taste
- Fresh herbs (such as parsley or thyme) for garnish (optional)

DIRECTIONS

- Preheat your grill to medium-high heat.
- Remove the outer leaves from the cauliflower and trim the stem end, leaving the core intact.
- Cut the cauliflower into 1-inch thick slices to create "steaks." You should be able to get 2-3 steaks from one head of cauliflower, depending on the size.
- In a small bowl, mix together the olive oil, minced garlic, paprika, cumin, salt, and pepper.
- Brush both sides of each cauliflower steak with the olive oil mixture.

NUTRITIONAL FACTS (PER SERVING)

- Calories: 80kcal
- Total Fat: 7g
- Saturated Fat: 1g
- Cholesterol: 0mg
- Sodium: 45mg
- Carbohydrates: 4g
- Dietary Fiber: 2g
- Sugars: 2g
- Protein: 2g

DIRECTIONS

- Place the cauliflower steaks on the preheated grill and cook for 5-6 minutes per side, or until tender and charred around the edges.
- Remove the cauliflower steaks from the grill and transfer them to a serving platter.
- Garnish with fresh herbs if desired and serve hot.

GRILLED SWORDFISH WITH HERB BUTTER

Prep Time 10 Mins

Cook Time 10 Mins

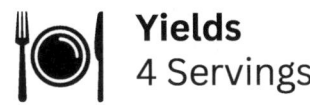

Yields 4 Servings

INGREDIENTS

- 4 swordfish steaks (about 6 ounces each)
- Salt and pepper to taste
- Cooking spray

For the Herb Butter:

- 4 tbsp unsalted butter, softened
- 2 tbsp chopped fresh herbs (such as parsley, dill, chives, or a combination)
- 1 clove garlic, minced
- 1 tsp lemon juice
- Salt and pepper to taste

DIRECTIONS

- Preheat your grill to medium-high heat.
- Season the swordfish steaks with salt and pepper on both sides.
- In a small bowl, combine the softened butter, chopped herbs, minced garlic, lemon juice, salt, and pepper. Mix until well combined.
- Grill the swordfish steaks for about 4-5 minutes per side, or until they are cooked through and have nice grill marks. The internal temperature should reach 145°F (63°C).
- While the swordfish is grilling, place a dollop of the herb butter on each steak.

NUTRITIONAL FACTS (PER SERVING)

- Calories: 270kcal
- Total Fat: 17g
- Saturated Fat: 8g
- Cholesterol: 130mg
- Sodium: 160mg
- Carbohydrates: 0g
- Dietary Fiber: 0g
- Sugars: 0g
- Protein: 26g

DIRECTIONS

- Once the swordfish is cooked, remove it from the grill and let it rest for a few minutes.
- Serve the grilled swordfish steaks with additional herb butter on top if desired.

GRILLED EGGPLANT SLICES

Prep Time
10 Mins

Cook Time
10 Mins

Yields
4 Servings

INGREDIENTS

- 1 large eggplant
- 2 tbsp olive oil
- 2 cloves garlic, minced (optional)
- Salt and pepper to taste
- Fresh herbs (such as parsley or basil), chopped for garnish (optional)

DIRECTIONS

- Preheat your grill to medium-high heat.
- Wash the eggplant and trim off the ends. Slice the eggplant into rounds, about 1/2 inch thick.
- In a small bowl, mix together the olive oil, minced garlic (if using), salt, and pepper.
- Brush both sides of the eggplant slices with the olive oil mixture.
- Place the eggplant slices directly onto the preheated grill.
- Grill the eggplant for 4-5 minutes on each side, or until tender and grill marks appear.
- Once cooked, remove the eggplant slices from the grill and transfer them to a serving platter.

NUTRITIONAL FACTS (PER SERVING)

- Calories: 60kcal
- Total Fat: 5g
- Saturated Fat: 1g
- Cholesterol: 0mg
- Sodium: 0mg
- Carbohydrates: 5g
- Dietary Fiber: 3g
- Sugars: 2g
- Protein: 1g

DIRECTIONS

- Garnish with fresh herbs if desired and serve hot.

GRILLED CHICKEN AND VEGGIE KABOBS

Prep Time 15 Mins

Cook Time 15 Mins

Yields 4 Servings

INGREDIENTS

- 1 lb boneless, skinless chicken breasts, cut into chunks
- 2 bell peppers (any color), cut into chunks
- 1 red onion, cut into chunks
- 1 zucchini, sliced
- 1 yellow squash, sliced
- Cherry tomatoes
- Wooden or metal skewers
- Salt and pepper to taste
- Optional marinade: lemon juice, olive oil, garlic, herbs (adjust to taste, but keep in mind the points if using oil)

DIRECTIONS

- If using wooden skewers, soak them in water for at least 30 minutes to prevent burning.
- In a bowl, combine the chicken chunks with the optional marinade ingredients, if using. Allow the chicken to marinate for at least 30 minutes in the refrigerator.
- Preheat your grill to medium-high heat.
- Thread the marinated chicken chunks, bell peppers, red onion, zucchini, yellow squash, and cherry tomatoes onto the skewers, alternating between ingredients.
- Season the assembled kabobs with salt and pepper to taste.

NUTRITIONAL FACTS (PER SERVING)

- Calories: 150kcal
- Total Fat: 3g
- Saturated Fat: 1g
- Cholesterol: 65mg
- Sodium: 60mg
- Carbohydrates: 8g
- Dietary Fiber: 2g
- Sugars: 4g
- Protein: 24g

DIRECTIONS

- Place the kabobs on the preheated grill and cook for about 10-15 minutes, turning occasionally, until the chicken is cooked through and the vegetables are tender and slightly charred.
- Once cooked, remove the kabobs from the grill and serve immediately.

GRILLED MAHI MAHI WITH MANGO SALSA

Prep Time 20 Mins
Cook Time 10 Mins
Yields 4 Servings

INGREDIENTS

For the Grilled Mahi Mahi:
- 4 Mahi Mahi fillets (about 6 ounces each)
- 2 tablespoons olive oil
- Salt and pepper to taste
- 1 teaspoon paprika
- 1 teaspoon garlic powder
- 1 teaspoon onion powder
- Juice of 1 lime

For the Mango Salsa:
- 2 ripe mangoes, diced
- 1/2 red onion, finely chopped
- 1 jalapeño pepper, seeded and finely chopped
- 1 red bell pepper, diced
- 1/4 cup fresh cilantro, chopped
- Juice of 2 limes
- Salt and pepper to taste

DIRECTIONS

- Preheat your grill to medium-high heat.
- In a small bowl, mix together the olive oil, salt, pepper, paprika, garlic powder, onion powder, and lime juice to create a marinade for the Mahi Mahi fillets.
- Place the Mahi Mahi fillets in a shallow dish and pour the marinade over them, ensuring they are evenly coated. Let them marinate for about 15-20 minutes while you prepare the salsa.
- In a separate bowl, combine the diced mangoes, red onion, jalapeño pepper, red bell pepper, cilantro, lime juice, salt, and pepper to make the mango salsa.

NUTRITIONAL FACTS (PER SERVING)

- Calories: 250kcal
- Total Fat: 9g
- Saturated Fat: 1.5g
- Cholesterol: 124mg
- Sodium: 100mg
- Carbohydrates: 17g
- Dietary Fiber: 3g
- Sugars: 12g
- Protein: 25g

DIRECTIONS

- Mix well and set aside.
- Once the grill is heated, grill the Mahi Mahi fillets for about 4-5 minutes on each side, or until they are cooked through and have grill marks. Cooking time may vary depending on the thickness of the fillets.
- Remove the grilled Mahi Mahi from the grill and serve hot, topped with the mango salsa.

GRILLED BELL PEPPER RINGS

Prep Time
5 Mins

Cook Time
10 Mins

Yields
4 Servings

INGREDIENTS

- 2 large bell peppers (any color), sliced into rings and seeds removed
- Cooking spray
- Salt and pepper to taste
- Optional: your choice of herbs or spices for seasoning (such as garlic powder, paprika, or Italian seasoning)

DIRECTIONS

- Preheat your grill to medium-high heat.
- Spray the bell pepper rings lightly with cooking spray on both sides.
- Season the bell pepper rings with salt, pepper, and any optional herbs or spices you prefer.
- Place the seasoned bell pepper rings directly onto the grill grates.
- Grill the bell pepper rings for about 4-5 minutes on each side, or until they are tender and have grill marks.
- Once done, remove the grilled bell pepper rings from the grill and serve immediately.

NUTRITIONAL FACTS (PER SERVING)

- Calories: 25kcal
- Total Fat: 0g
- Saturated Fat: 0g
- Cholesterol: 0mg
- Sodium: 1mg
- Carbohydrates: 6g
- Dietary Fiber: 2g
- Sugars: 3g
- Protein: 1g

GRILLED TURKEY SAUSAGES

Prep Time
10 Mins

Cook Time
12 Mins

Yields
6 turkey sausages

INGREDIENTS

- 1 pound lean ground turkey
- 2 cloves garlic, minced
- 1 teaspoon fennel seeds
- 1 teaspoon paprika
- 1 teaspoon dried oregano
- 1/2 teaspoon salt
- 1/2 teaspoon black pepper
- Cooking spray

DIRECTIONS

- In a large mixing bowl, combine the ground turkey, minced garlic, fennel seeds, paprika, dried oregano, salt, and black pepper. Mix until well combined.
- Divide the mixture into equal portions and shape them into sausage patties or links.
- Preheat your grill to medium-high heat.
- Spray the grill grates with cooking spray to prevent sticking.
- Place the turkey sausages on the preheated grill and cook for 5-6 minutes on each side, or until they are cooked through and reach an internal temperature of 165°F (75°C).

NUTRITIONAL FACTS (PER SERVING)

- Calories: 100kcal
- Total Fat: 6g
- Saturated Fat: 2g
- Cholesterol: 55mg
- Sodium: 280mg
- Carbohydrates: 1g
- Dietary Fiber: 0g
- Sugars: 0g
- Protein: 10g

DIRECTIONS

- Once cooked, remove the sausages from the grill and let them rest for a few minutes before serving.

GRILLED BRUSCHETTA CHICKEN

Prep Time 10 Mins

Cook Time 15 Mins

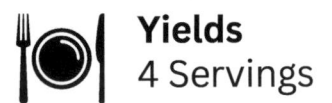

Yields 4 Servings

INGREDIENTS

- 4 boneless, skinless chicken breasts
- 4 medium tomatoes, diced
- 2 cloves garlic, minced
- 1/4 cup fresh basil, chopped
- 1 tablespoon balsamic vinegar
- Salt and pepper to taste
- Cooking spray or olive oil for grilling.

DIRECTIONS

- Preheat your grill to medium-high heat.
- In a mixing bowl, combine diced tomatoes, minced garlic, chopped basil, and balsamic vinegar. Season with salt and pepper to taste. Set aside.
- Season the chicken breasts with salt and pepper on both sides.
- Grill the chicken breasts for about 6-7 minutes on each side, or until cooked through and no longer pink in the center.
- Once the chicken is cooked, top each breast with a generous spoonful of the tomato mixture.
- Serve immediately.

**NUTRITIONAL FACTS
(PER SERVING)**

- Calories: 170kcal
- Total Fat: 3g
- Saturated Fat: 1g
- Cholesterol: 73mg
- Sodium: 80mg
- Carbohydrates: 6g
- Dietary Fiber: 2g
- Sugars: 4g
- Protein: 29g

GRILLED RADICCHIO WEDGES

Prep Time
10 Mins

Cook Time
10 Mins

Yields
8 Servings

INGREDIENTS

- 2 heads of radicchio, each cut into 4 wedges
- 2 tablespoons balsamic vinegar
- 1 tablespoon olive oil
- Salt and pepper to taste
- Optional toppings: grated Parmesan cheese, chopped fresh herbs (such as parsley or thyme)

DIRECTIONS

- Preheat your grill to medium-high heat.
- In a small bowl, whisk together the balsamic vinegar and olive oil to create a marinade.
- Brush the radicchio wedges with the marinade, coating them evenly on all sides. Season with salt and pepper to taste.
- Place the radicchio wedges on the preheated grill and cook for 3-4 minutes per side, or until they are slightly charred and tender.
- Remove the grilled radicchio wedges from the grill and transfer them to a serving platter.

NUTRITIONAL FACTS (PER SERVING)

- Calories: 20kcal
- Total Fat: 1g
- Saturated Fat: 0g
- Cholesterol: 0mg
- Sodium: 10mg
- Carbohydrates: 3g
- Dietary Fiber: 1g
- Sugars: 1g
- Protein: 1g

DIRECTIONS

- If desired, sprinkle the grilled radicchio wedges with grated Parmesan cheese and chopped fresh herbs before serving.

GRILLED CHICKEN FAJITAS

Prep Time
10 Mins

Cook Time
15 Mins

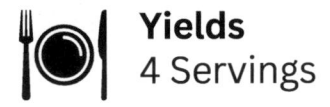

Yields
4 Servings

INGREDIENTS

- 1 lb boneless, skinless chicken breasts
- 3 bell peppers (any combination of colors), sliced
- 1 large onion, sliced
- 2 cloves garlic, minced
- 2 tbsp fajita seasoning (store-bought or homemade)
- Juice of 1 lime
- Salt and pepper to taste
- Cooking spray

DIRECTIONS

- Marinate chicken in fajita seasoning, garlic, lime juice, salt, and pepper for at least 30 minutes.
- Preheat grill to medium-high heat, then grill chicken for 6-8 minutes per side until cooked through.
- Let chicken rest, then slice thinly against the grain.
- In a skillet, cook sliced bell peppers and onions until tender and slightly caramelized.
- Combine cooked chicken with peppers and onions in the skillet.

NUTRITIONAL FACTS (PER SERVING)

- Calories: 200kcal
- Total Fat: 3g
- Saturated Fat: 1g
- Cholesterol: 96mg
- Sodium: 230mg
- Carbohydrates: 10g
- Dietary Fiber: 3g
- Sugars: 5g
- Protein: 33g

DIRECTIONS

- Serve with optional toppings such as salsa, guacamole, Greek yogurt, shredded lettuce, chopped tomatoes, shredded cheese, and whole wheat tortillas or lettuce wraps.

GRILLED FISH TACOS

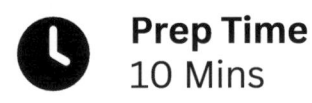

Prep Time
10 Mins

Cook Time
8 Mins

Yields
4 Servings

INGREDIENTS

- 1 pound white fish fillets (such as tilapia, cod, or halibut)
- 1 tablespoon olive oil
- 1 teaspoon chili powder
- 1 teaspoon cumin
- 1/2 teaspoon paprika
- Salt and pepper to taste
- 8 small corn tortillas
- Optional toppings: shredded cabbage, sliced avocado, diced tomatoes, cilantro, lime wedges

DIRECTIONS

- **Prepare the Tzatziki Sauce:** In a bowl, combine the Greek yogurt, grated cucumber, minced garlic, lemon juice, olive oil, and chopped dill.
- Mix well until all ingredients are fully incorporated.
- Season with salt and pepper to taste. Adjust seasoning if needed.
- Refrigerate the tzatziki sauce for at least 30 minutes to allow the flavors to meld.
- **Slice the Cucumbers:** Wash and dry the remaining cucumbers.
- Using a sharp knife or a mandoline slicer, thinly slice the cucumbers into rounds.

NUTRITIONAL FACTS (PER SERVING)

- Calories: 150kcal
- Protein: 20g
- Fat: 4g
- Carbohydrates: 10g
- Fiber: 2g
- Sugar: 0g

DIRECTIONS

- **Assemble:** Arrange the cucumber slices on a serving platter.
- Spoon the prepared tzatziki sauce over the cucumber slices, or serve it on the side as a dipping sauce.
- Garnish with fresh dill or mint leaves, if desired.
- **Serve:** Serve the sliced cucumbers with tzatziki sauce immediately as a refreshing appetizer or snack.

GRILLED PORK TENDERLOIN

Prep Time 10 Mins **Cook Time** 20 Mins **Yields** 4 Servings

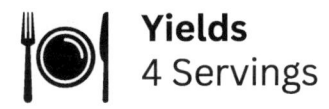

INGREDIENTS

- 1 lb pork tenderloin
- 2 cloves garlic, minced
- 1 tablespoon fresh rosemary, chopped
- 1 tablespoon fresh thyme, chopped
- 1 tablespoon fresh parsley, chopped
- 1 teaspoon paprika
- 1 teaspoon salt
- 1/2 teaspoon black pepper
- Cooking spray or olive oil spray

DIRECTIONS

- In a small bowl, mix together minced garlic, chopped rosemary, thyme, parsley, paprika, salt, and black pepper to create a marinade rub.
- Rub the marinade mixture all over the pork tenderloin, ensuring it's evenly coated. Let it marinate for at least 30 minutes, or overnight in the refrigerator for maximum flavor.
- Preheat your grill to medium-high heat.
- Lightly coat the grill grates with cooking spray or olive oil spray to prevent sticking.
- Place the marinated pork tenderloin on the grill and cook for about 15-20 minutes, turning occasionally,

NUTRITIONAL FACTS (PER SERVING)

- Calories: 160kcal
- Total Fat: 4g
- Saturated Fat: 1g
- Cholesterol: 75mg
- Sodium: 610mg
- Carbohydrates: 1g
- Dietary Fiber: 0g
- Sugars: 0g
- Protein: 28g

DIRECTIONS

- until the internal temperature reaches 145°F (63°C) for medium-rare or up to 160°F (71°C) for medium, using a meat thermometer to check for doneness.
- Once cooked to your desired level, remove the pork tenderloin from the grill and let it rest for a few minutes before slicing.
- Slice the grilled pork tenderloin into thin slices and serve hot.

GRILLED CAPRESE CHICKEN

Prep Time
10 Mins

Cook Time
15 Mins

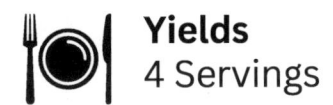

Yields
4 Servings

INGREDIENTS

- 4 boneless, skinless chicken breasts
- 2 large tomatoes, sliced
- 4 slices fresh mozzarella cheese
- 1/4 cup fresh basil leaves
- 2 cloves garlic, minced
- 2 tablespoons balsamic vinegar
- 1 tablespoon olive oil
- Salt and pepper to taste

DIRECTIONS

- Preheat your grill to medium-high heat.
- Season the chicken breasts with salt, pepper, and minced garlic.
- Place the chicken breasts on the preheated grill and cook for 6-8 minutes per side, or until they are cooked through and have grill marks.
- While the chicken is cooking, place the tomato slices on the grill and cook for 2-3 minutes per side, or until they are slightly charred.
- Once the chicken is cooked, remove it from the grill and top each breast with a slice of mozzarella cheese. Allow the cheese to melt slightly.

NUTRITIONAL FACTS (PER SERVING)

- Calories: 250kcal
- Total Fat: 10g
- Saturated Fat: 3.5g
- Cholesterol: 90mg
- Sodium: 210mg
- Carbohydrates: 4g
- Dietary Fiber: 1g
- Sugars: 2g
- Protein: 35g

DIRECTIONS

- To assemble, place a grilled tomato slice on top of each chicken breast, followed by fresh basil leaves.
- Drizzle the balsamic vinegar and olive oil over the top of each chicken breast.
- Serve immediately.

GRILLED TILAPIA WITH LEMON BUTTER

Prep Time
5 Mins

Cook Time
8 Mins

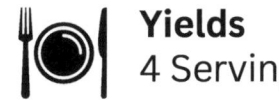

Yields
4 Servings

INGREDIENTS

- 4 tilapia fillets
- 2 tablespoons unsalted butter
- 2 tablespoons fresh lemon juice
- 2 cloves garlic, minced
- Salt and pepper to taste
- Lemon slices for garnish
- Chopped parsley for garnish (optional)

DIRECTIONS

- Preheat your grill to medium-high heat.
- In a small saucepan, melt the butter over low heat.
- Stir in the minced garlic and cook for 1-2 minutes until fragrant.
- Remove the saucepan from the heat and stir in the fresh lemon juice. Set aside.
- Season both sides of the tilapia fillets with salt and pepper.
- Place the seasoned tilapia fillets on the preheated grill.
- Grill the tilapia for 3-4 minutes on each side, or until cooked through and easily flaked with a fork.

NUTRITIONAL FACTS (PER SERVING)

- Calories: 145kcal
- Total Fat: 7g
- Saturated Fat: 3g
- Cholesterol: 59mg
- Sodium: 68mg
- Carbohydrates: 1g
- Dietary Fiber: 0g
- Sugars: 0g
- Protein: 20g

DIRECTIONS

- During the last minute of cooking, brush the lemon butter mixture over the tilapia fillets.
- Remove the tilapia from the grill and transfer to a serving platter.
- Garnish with lemon slices and chopped parsley, if desired.
- Serve hot and enjoy.

GRILLED GREEK CHICKEN SOUVLAKI

Prep Time
40 Mins

Cook Time
14 Mins

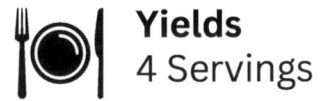

Yields
4 Servings

INGREDIENTS

- 1 lb boneless, skinless chicken breasts, cut into bite-sized pieces
- 2 cloves garlic, minced
- 2 tbsp lemon juice
- 1 tbsp olive oil
- 1 tsp dried oregano
- 1/2 tsp dried thyme
- 1/2 tsp dried rosemary
- Salt and pepper to taste
- Wooden skewers, soaked in water for 30 minutes

DIRECTIONS

- In a large bowl, combine the minced garlic, lemon juice, olive oil, dried oregano, dried thyme, dried rosemary, salt, and pepper. Mix well to create the marinade.
- Add the chicken pieces to the marinade and toss until evenly coated. Cover the bowl and refrigerate for at least 30 minutes to marinate, or up to 4 hours for best flavor.
- Preheat the grill to medium-high heat.
- Thread the marinated chicken pieces onto the soaked wooden skewers.
- Place the skewers on the preheated grill and cook for 5-7 minutes on each side,

NUTRITIONAL FACTS (PER SERVING)

- Calories: 140kcal
- Total Fat: 4g
- Saturated Fat: 1g
- Cholesterol: 65mg
- Sodium: 70mg
- Carbohydrates: 1g
- Dietary Fiber: 0g
- Sugars: 0g
- Protein: 25g

DIRECTIONS

- or until the chicken is cooked through and has grill marks.
- Once cooked, remove the skewers from the grill and let them rest for a few minutes before serving.
- Serve the Grilled Greek Chicken Souvlaki with your favorite sides, such as Greek salad, tzatziki sauce, pita bread, or grilled vegetables.

GRILLED CABBAGE WEDGES

Prep Time
10 Mins

Cook Time
14 Mins

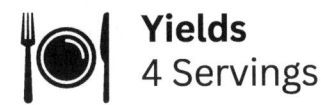

Yields
4 Servings

INGREDIENTS

- 1 head of cabbage
- Olive oil spray
- Salt and pepper to taste
- Optional: Garlic powder, onion powder, paprika, or any other desired seasonings.

DIRECTIONS

- Preheat your grill to medium-high heat.
- Cut the cabbage into wedges, leaving the core intact to hold the wedges together.
- Spray the cabbage wedges lightly with olive oil spray on both sides.
- Season the cabbage wedges with salt, pepper, and any other desired seasonings.
- Place the cabbage wedges on the preheated grill, directly over the heat.
- Grill the cabbage wedges for about 5-7 minutes per side, or until they are tender and charred in spots.
- Remove the grilled cabbage wedges from the grill and serve hot.

**NUTRITIONAL FACTS
(PER SERVING)**

- Calories: 35kcal
- Total Fat: 0g
- Saturated Fat: 0g
- Cholesterol: 0mg
- Sodium: 26mg
- Carbohydrates: 8g
- Dietary Fiber: 4g
- Sugars: 4g
- Protein: 2g

GRILLED TERIYAKI TOFU

Prep Time
15 Mins

Cook Time
10 Mins

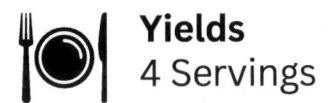

Yields
4 Servings

INGREDIENTS

- 1 block (14 oz) extra firm tofu, drained and pressed
- 1/2 cup soy sauce (use reduced-sodium for a healthier option)
- 1/4 cup water
- 2 tablespoons rice vinegar
- 2 tablespoons honey or maple syrup (or a sugar substitute for a lower-calorie option)
- 2 cloves garlic, minced
- 1 teaspoon grated fresh ginger
- 1 tablespoon cornstarch (optional, for thickening the sauce)
- Cooking spray or oil for grilling.

DIRECTIONS

- Prepare the tofu by draining it and pressing it to remove excess moisture. You can do this by wrapping the tofu block in a clean kitchen towel or paper towels and placing a heavy object on top for about 15-20 minutes.
- In a small saucepan, combine the soy sauce, water, rice vinegar, honey or maple syrup, minced garlic, and grated ginger. Bring the mixture to a simmer over medium heat.
- If you prefer a thicker sauce, mix the cornstarch with a little water to create a slurry. Slowly add the slurry to the sauce while whisking constantly until it thickens slightly.

NUTRITIONAL FACTS (PER SERVING)

- Calories: 110kcal
- Total Fat: 4g
- Saturated Fat: 0.5g
- Cholesterol: 0mg
- Carbohydrates: 10g
- Dietary Fiber: 1g
- Sugars: 5g
- Protein: 9g

DIRECTIONS

- Remove from heat and let it cool. Cut the pressed tofu into slices or cubes, depending on your preference.
- Place the tofu in a shallow dish and pour half of the teriyaki sauce over it, reserving the other half for later. Allow the tofu to marinate for at least 15-30 minutes, turning occasionally to ensure even coating.
- Preheat your grill or grill pan over medium-high heat and lightly grease the surface with cooking spray or oil.
- Grill the marinated tofu for about 3-4 minutes on each side, or until lightly browned and heated through, basting with the remaining teriyaki sauce as desired.
- Once grilled, remove the tofu from the grill and let it rest for a few minutes before serving.

GRILLED VEGETABLE QUESADILLAS

Prep Time
10 Mins

Cook Time
15 Mins

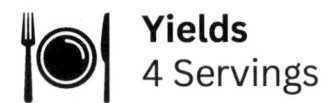

Yields
4 Servings

INGREDIENTS

- 1 medium zucchini, sliced
- 1 medium yellow squash, sliced
- 1 red bell pepper, sliced
- 1 green bell pepper, sliced
- 1 medium onion, sliced
- 4 whole wheat tortillas (8-inch)
- 1 cup fat-free shredded cheddar cheese
- Cooking spray
- Salt and pepper to taste
- Optional toppings: salsa, non-fat Greek yogurt or sour cream, chopped cilantro.

DIRECTIONS

- Preheat grill or grill pan over medium-high heat.
- Spray the grill or grill pan with cooking spray.
- Place the sliced zucchini, yellow squash, bell peppers, and onion on the grill.
- Grill the vegetables for 4-5 minutes on each side, or until tender and lightly charred.
- Remove the grilled vegetables from the grill and season with salt and pepper to taste.
- Lay out the tortillas and divide the grilled vegetables evenly among them, placing them on one half of each tortilla.
- Sprinkle each tortilla with 1/4 cup of fat-free shredded cheddar cheese.

NUTRITIONAL FACTS (PER SERVING)

- Calories: 150kcal
- Total Fat: 1.5g
- Saturated Fat: 0g
- Cholesterol: 0mg
- Sodium: 250mg
- Carbohydrates: 28g
- Dietary Fiber: 5g
- Sugars: 6g
- Protein: 10g

DIRECTIONS

- Fold the tortillas in half over the filling to form quesadillas.
- Spray the grill or grill pan with cooking spray again and place the quesadillas on the grill.
- Grill the quesadillas for 2-3 minutes on each side, or until golden brown and the cheese is melted.
- Remove the quesadillas from the grill and let them cool slightly before slicing into wedges.
- Serve hot with optional toppings such as salsa, non-fat Greek yogurt or sour cream, and chopped cilantro.

GRILLED VEGETABLE PLATTER WITH HUMMUS

Prep Time 15 Mins   **Cook Time** 10 Mins   **Yields** 4 Servings

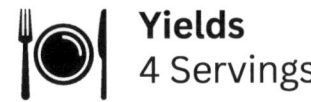

INGREDIENTS

- Assorted vegetables (such as bell peppers, zucchini, eggplant, cherry tomatoes, and mushrooms), washed and sliced
- 1 tablespoon olive oil
- Salt and pepper to taste
- 1 cup of plain non-fat Greek yogurt
- 1 tablespoon lemon juice
- 2 cloves garlic, minced
- 1 teaspoon ground cumin
- 1 teaspoon paprika
- Salt and pepper to taste
- Fresh parsley for garnish (optional)

DIRECTIONS

- Preheat your grill to medium-high heat.
- In a large bowl, toss the sliced vegetables with olive oil, salt, and pepper until evenly coated.
- Place the vegetables on the grill and cook for 4-5 minutes on each side, or until they are tender and have grill marks.
- While the vegetables are grilling, prepare the hummus. In a medium bowl, combine the Greek yogurt, lemon juice, minced garlic, ground cumin, paprika, salt, and pepper. Stir until well combined.
- Once the vegetables are grilled to your liking, remove them from the grill and arrange them on a serving platter.

NUTRITIONAL FACTS (PER SERVING)

- Calories: 80kcal
- Total Fat: 4g
- Saturated Fat: 0.5g
- Cholesterol: 0mg
- Sodium: 25mg
- Carbohydrates: 7g
- Dietary Fiber: 2g
- Sugars: 4g
- Protein: 6g

DIRECTIONS

- Garnish the hummus with fresh parsley, if desired.
- Serve the grilled vegetables with the hummus on the side for dipping.

GRILLED SPICY TOFU

Prep Time
40 Mins

Cook Time
14 Mins

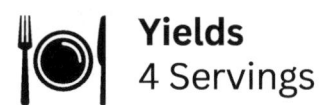

Yields
4 Servings

including marinating

INGREDIENTS

- 1 block (about 14 oz) extra-firm tofu, pressed and drained
- 2 tbsp soy sauce or tamari
- 1 tbsp sriracha sauce (adjust according to your spice preference)
- 1 tbsp lime juice
- 1 clove garlic, minced
- 1 tsp ground cumin
- 1 tsp paprika
- 1/2 tsp chili powder
- Cooking spray or oil for greasing the grill

DIRECTIONS

- Begin by pressing the tofu to remove excess water. Place the block of tofu between two clean kitchen towels or paper towels and place a heavy object on top (such as a skillet or a stack of plates). Let it press for about 20-30 minutes.
- While the tofu is pressing, prepare the marinade. In a small bowl, whisk together the soy sauce, sriracha sauce, lime juice, minced garlic, cumin, paprika, and chili powder.
- Once the tofu is pressed, slice it into your desired thickness, keeping in mind that thinner slices will absorb more flavor.

NUTRITIONAL FACTS (PER SERVING)

- Calories: 100kcal
- Total Fat: 5g
- Saturated Fat: 0.5g
- Cholesterol: 0mg
- Sodium: 480mg
- Carbohydrates: 5g
- Dietary Fiber: 1g
- Sugars: 1g
- Protein: 10g

DIRECTIONS

- Place the tofu slices in a shallow dish or a resealable plastic bag, and pour the marinade over them. Ensure all slices are coated evenly. Marinate for at least 30 minutes, or longer for more flavor.
- Preheat your grill or grill pan over medium-high heat. Lightly grease the grill grates with cooking spray or oil to prevent sticking.
- Once the grill is hot, place the tofu slices on the grill. Cook for about 5-7 minutes on each side, or until grill marks form and the tofu is heated through.
- Remove the tofu from the grill and serve hot. You can garnish with chopped cilantro or green onions if desired.

GRILLED BUFFALO CAULIFLOWER

Prep Time
10 Mins

Cook Time
15 Mins

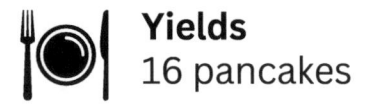

Yields
16 pancakes

INGREDIENTS

- 1 large head of cauliflower, cut into florets
- 1/4 cup hot sauce (such as Frank's RedHot)
- 2 tablespoons olive oil
- 1 teaspoon garlic powder
- 1 teaspoon onion powder
- Salt and pepper, to taste
- Ranch or blue cheese dressing for dipping (optional)

DIRECTIONS

- In a large mixing bowl, mash the bananas until smooth.
- Add the eggs to the mashed bananas and whisk until well combined. You can also add vanilla extract at this stage if desired.
- Heat a non-stick skillet or griddle over medium heat. Lightly grease the surface with cooking spray or butter.
- Pour the pancake batter onto the skillet to form pancakes of desired size (about 1/4 cup of batter for each pancake).
- Cook the pancakes for 2-3 minutes on one side, or until bubbles begin to form on the surface.

NUTRITIONAL FACTS (PER SERVING)

- Calories: 65kcal
- Total Fat: 2g
- Saturated Fat: 1g
- Cholesterol: 93mg
- Sodium: 32mg
- Carbohydrates: 8g
- Dietary Fiber: 1g
- Sugars: 5g
- Protein: 4g

DIRECTIONS

- Flip the pancakes and cook for an additional 1-2 minutes on the other side, or until golden brown and cooked through.
- Repeat with the remaining batter, greasing the skillet as needed between batches.

Meal plan
for 30 Days

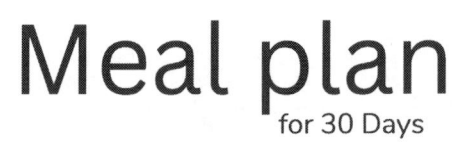

Date: _____

	BREAKFAST	LUNCH	DINNER
MON	Scrambled eggs with spinach and tomatoes	Grilled chicken breast with a mixed green salad (lettuce, cucumber, bell peppers) and balsamic vinaigrette	Baked salmon with steamed broccoli and cauliflower
TUE	Greek yogurt with fresh berries and a sprinkle of chia seeds	Turkey lettuce wraps with hummus and sliced veggies	Stir-fried shrimp with bell peppers, onions, and zucchini served over cauliflower rice
WED	Oatmeal topped with sliced banana and a dollop of almond butter	Quinoa salad with cherry tomatoes, cucumber, red onion, and lemon-tahini dressing	Grilled tofu with roasted Brussels sprouts and carrots
THU	Veggie omelet (with mushrooms, onions, bell peppers) cooked in olive oil	Lentil soup with a side of mixed greens dressed with lemon juice	Baked cod with asparagus and a side of mixed bean salad
FRI	Smoothie made with spinach, frozen berries, banana, and almond milk	Grilled shrimp skewers with a side of Greek salad (tomatoes, cucumbers, olives, feta cheese)	Zucchini noodles with marinara sauce and grilled chicken breast
SAT	Cottage cheese topped with pineapple chunks and a sprinkle of cinnamon	Tuna salad lettuce wraps with diced celery and carrots	Turkey chili with black beans, diced tomatoes, and bell peppers

Meal plan
for 30 Days

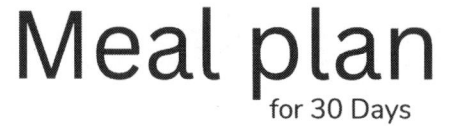

Date _____

	BREAKFAST	LUNCH	DINNER
SUN	Whole grain toast with mashed avocado and sliced tomato	Egg salad stuffed in bell pepper halves served with a side of carrot sticks	Grilled steak with roasted green beans and a side of quinoa

Week 2-4

- Continue to repeat and vary these meal ideas throughout the 30-day period, incorporating a wide range of fruits, vegetables, lean proteins, and whole grains. Remember to drink plenty of water throughout the day.

ZERO POINT FOOD LIST

Zero Point Fruits
- Apples
- Apricots
- Bananas
- Blackberries
- Blueberries
- Cantaloupe
- Cherries
- Clementine
- Coconut
- Cranberries
- Dates
- Dragon Fruit
- Figs
- Grapefruit
- Grapes (any variety)
- Guava
- Honeydew Melon
- Jackfruit
- Kiwi
- Lemon
- Lime
- Mango
- Oranges
- Passion Fruit
- Peach
- Pears
- Pineapple

BEANS & LEGUMES
- Adzuki beans
- Alfalfa sprouts
- Bean sprouts
- Black beans
- Black-eyed peas
- Cannellini beans
- Chickpeas
- Edamame
- Fava beans
- Great Northern beans
- Hominy
- Kidney beans
- Lentils
- Lima beans
- Lupini beans
- Navy beans
- Pinto beans
- Refried beans, canned, fat-free
- Soy beans

CHICKEN & TURKEY BREAST
- Ground chicken breast
- Ground turkey, 98% fat-free
- Ground turkey breast
- Skinless chicken breast
- Skinless turkey breast

EGGS
- Egg substitute
- Egg whites
- Egg yolks
- Eggs

Zero Point Vegetables (Starchy & Non-Starchy)
- Arrowroot, raw
- Artichoke
- Arugula
- Asparagus
- Broccoli
- Beans (black, adzuki, cannellini, garbanzo, kidney, great northern, lima, pinto, etc.)
- Beans, refried (canned, fat-free, no added sugar)
- Green Beans
- Bok Choy
- Brussel Sprouts
- Cabbage
- Carrots
- Cauliflower
- Celery
- Chard
- Chickpeas
- Collards
- Corn
- Cucumber
- Daikon
- Edamame
- Eggplant
- Endive
- Fennel
- Ginger Root
- Kale
- Leeks
- Lettuce (any variety)
- Mushrooms
- Okra
- Peas
- Peppers (bell)
- Pickles (without sugar)
- Pumpkin
- Radishes
- Scallions (green onions)
- Spinach
- Sprouts
- Squash
- Tomatoes
- Turnips
- Zucchini

Zero Point Herbs and Spices
- Basil
- Chives
- Cinnamon
- Dill Weed
- Garlic
- Garlic Salt
- Italian Seasoning
- Oregano
- Paprika
- Parsley
- Pepper
- Peppermint
- Pumpkin Spice
- Rosemary
- Sage
- Salt
- Thyme

Zero Point Meat, Seafood and Poultry
- Calamari, grilled
- Chicken Breast (boneless, skinless)
- Crab (Alaska king, Dungeness, queen, king)
- Crayfish
- Eggs
- Bass Fish
- Bluefish
- Carp
- Catfish
- Cod
- Eel
- Grouper
- Haddock
- Halibut
- Lobster
- Mackerel Fish
- Mussels
- Octopus
- Oysters
- Salmon (Atlantic and farm raised)
- Sardines
- Sea Bass
- Shrimp
- Sturgeon Fish
- Swordfish
- Tilapia Fish

FISH/SHELLFISH
- Abalone
- Alaskan king crab
- Anchovies, in water
- Arctic char
- Bluefish
- Branzino
- Butterfish
- Canned tuna, in water
- Carp
- Catfish
- Caviar
- Clams
- Cod
- Crabmeat, lump
- Crayfish
- Cuttlefish
- Dungeness crab
- Eel
- Fish roe
- Flounder
- Grouper
- Haddock
- Halibut
- Herring
- Lobster
- Mahi mahi
- Monkfish
- Mussels
- Octopus
- Orange roughy
- Oysters
- Perch
- Pike
- Pollock
- Pompano
- Salmon
- Sardines, canned in water or sauce
- Sashimi
- Scallops
- Sea bass
- Sea cucumber
- Sea urchin
- Shrimp
- Smelt
- Smoked haddock
- Smoked salmon
- Smoked sturgeon
- Smoked trout
- Smoked whitefish
- Snails
- Snapper
- Sole
- Squid

Zero Point Drinks
- Water
- Coffee, black (without sugar)
- Coke Zero (all varieties)
- Diet Coke (all varieties)
- Fresca (all varieties)
- Gatorade Zero
- Sparkling Ice Water (all flavors)
- Tea, black
- Vitamin Water Zero

Zero Point Snacks
- Applesauce, unsweetened
- Fruit cup (canned in water pack, no sugar added)
- Fruit cup (fresh)
- Vegetable Sticks
- Yogurt (greek, plain, fat-free, unsweetened)

Made in the USA
Las Vegas, NV
09 March 2024

86953673R00046